Badiane Ousseyne
Mangane Abdoulaye
Thierno Taibou Diallo

Evaluation of the national covid vaccine deployment plan

Badiane Ousseyne
Mangane Abdoulaye
Thierno Taibou Diallo

Evaluation of the national covid vaccine deployment plan

ScienciaScripts

Imprint

Any brand names and product names mentioned in this book are subject to trademark, brand or patent protection and are trademarks or registered trademarks of their respective holders. The use of brand names, product names, common names, trade names, product descriptions etc. even without a particular marking in this work is in no way to be construed to mean that such names may be regarded as unrestricted in respect of trademark and brand protection legislation and could thus be used by anyone.

Cover image: www.ingimage.com

This book is a translation from the original published under ISBN 978-620-6-71710-2.

Publisher:
Sciencia Scripts
is a trademark of
Dodo Books Indian Ocean Ltd. and OmniScriptum S.R.L publishing group

120 High Road, East Finchley, London, N2 9ED, United Kingdom
Str. Armeneasca 28/1, office 1, Chisinau MD-2012, Republic of Moldova, Europe
Printed at: see last page
ISBN: 978-620-7-91185-1

ACKNOWLEDGEMENTS

I thank Allah, the Almighty, the Clement and the Merciful, who has eternal power over me. Thanks to Him, we have come this far.

To my supervisors at the Senegal Prevention Department *(Dr Ousseynou Badiane, Abdoulaye Mangane, Youssouf M'baye and Ibrahima Mbaye): for your availability, your welcome and the advice you gave me, all of which will be useful in my professional career. Right from the start, I felt I was in a familiar environment. Allow me to say a big thank you. May God give you long life.*

To my thesis sponsor, Dr Marie-Laure KLEME: *you kindly agreed to be the sponsor of this work and to supervise it despite your busy schedule. Your scientific quality and your unconditional availability meant that I was able to achieve the results I had hoped for. More than a master, you have been an advisor. Dear Master, allow me to reiterate my deep gratitude. May God perpetuate your work throughout the world and bring prosperity and health to your family.*

To Professor René Migliani: *thank you for taking your precious time to enrich my work. Please accept my sincere gratitude.*

To the auditors of the health department at Senghor University *(Amadou Oury Diallo, Zinsou Rodrigue Ahodegnon, Nambinintsoa Lima Rose and Nehemie Phycien): you have contributed to the development of this jewel by providing me with excellent guidelines. May God guide your steps and crown you with full success in your activities. Allow me simply to say thank you.*

To the 18th graduating class of Senghor University: *my time with you has been a wonderful experience. I have learned to live in a multicultural community that will remain engraved in my memory.*

To my colleagues and collaborators in Guinea's Expanded Programme on Immunisation *(Dr Ibrahima Somparé, Idrissa Baldé and Dr Kalissa Sakoba): I would like to take this opportunity to express my gratitude and appreciation. From afar, you have never ceased to bless me, encourage me and give me advice.*

To my family: *it's an unforgettable day for me to be able to put into practice the effort you have made for me during my studies. I can't mention any names here, but I want you to know that you have all played an important role in helping me to achieve my goal. May God bless you, give you long life and cast his shadow over you and your children. May God strengthen the bonds of kinship between all the members and help me to remain grateful to you.*

DEDICATION

To my late father Thierno Ibrahima DIALLO"BABA", *here I am taking a step forward without you physically, and yet you have been the architect of this journey. Your passion for health has made me what I am today. Thank you, Dad, for everything you've done for me. Rest in peace. May God give us the faith and strength to complete your mission.*

To my Mother Hadja Kadiatou BALDE, a *courageous, combative and generous Mother. This is the long-awaited moment that will see the crowning of your support. Thank you "Néné", may God give you long life.*

To my brothers and sisters, *today is an unforgettable day for me, because I've been able to make good on the effort you've made during my studies. You promised to support me in my studies and you have done so. This work is also yours.*

To my *understanding* **husband Amadou DIALLO,** *here we are at the end of the work we have undertaken together. You have supported me morally and psychologically. Thank you and I will be eternally grateful.*

To my children (Fatoumata Lamarana, Oumar Bella, Abdoulaye Sadio and Aissatou Sélé DIALLO), *I am proud today to dedicate this work to you. I had to miss some historic moments in your lives, but it was necessary and I invite you to follow this fine example. May God illuminate your path to school and give you long life.*

To the Senghor 18 Guinean community, *together we have formed a lovely family and you have accepted my title of "Diadia" which I love very much. Please accept my sincere gratitude.*

SUMMARY

Introduction: Post-introduction evaluation **of** vaccines is standard practice in the Expanded Programme on Immunisation within the healthcare system. It must be carried out within a well-defined period of time, between 6 and 18 months after the start of vaccination. Senegal introduced Covid-19 vaccines into its immunisation programme through a national Covid-19 vaccine deployment plan on 26 February 2021. To the best of our knowledge, no assessment has yet been carried out to evaluate the Covid-19 vaccine deployment plan in Senegal's Expanded Programme on Immunisation. This work has enabled us to assess the situation two years after the deployment of these vaccines.

Methods: This was a cross-sectional evaluative study carried out from 2 to 14 July 2023 in the Dakar medical region at all levels of the health pyramid, with stakeholders involved in vaccination (Prevention Directorate, Dakar medical region, three health districts and 8 vaccination sites) to assess the preparation and implementation of the national plan for the deployment of Covid-19 vaccines in Senegal's vaccination programme.

Results: A total of 13 sites involved in vaccination against Covid-19 were visited. The area of regulatory preparation carried out by the central level was 100% implemented. On the other hand, weak achievements were noted in the following areas

- planning and coordination of vaccine introduction at district level (0% for regular technical group meetings) ;

- Acceptance and uptake of vaccination (38% of local social mobilisation activities organised specifically for the Covid-19 vaccine and 0% of posters displayed at vaccination sites);

- Vaccine safety monitoring, management of post-vaccination adverse events (AEFIs) and serious adverse events (0% coverage of all AEFIs for vaccination against Covid-19).

This study enabled us to confirm that the national Covid-19 vaccine deployment plan was effective using the usual vaccination system. However, there were shortcomings in the implementation of these activities, such as communication and social mobilisation, and the management of MAPI.

Keywords Covid-19, Dakar, Post-introduction, Routine vaccination

TABLE OF CONTENTS

1 INTRODUCTION

Covid-19 is a zoonosis caused by the severe acute respiratory syndrome coronavirus 2 (SARS-CoV-2) [1]. This virus causes respiratory tract infections ranging from the common cold to severe respiratory distress syndrome. It is generally spread by inhalation of droplets produced by coughing or sneezing, or by contact with the mucous membranes of the mouth, nose and eyes [2]. Initially discovered in the city of Wuhan in China in December 2019, Covid-19 assumed pandemic proportions in the early months of 2020. The first case on the African continent was diagnosed in Egypt on 25 February 2020[3].

As of 21 February 2023, the World Health Organisation (WHO) reported 757,264,511 confirmed cases, including 6,850,594 deaths. Worldwide vaccination coverage for the 1ère dose was 64.93% [4].

Mortality from Covid-19 was higher in the elderly, healthcare workers and people with co-morbidities [5]. The major complication is respiratory. Late complications such as pulmonary fibrosis, venous thromboembolism, arterial thrombosis, cardiac thrombosis and inflammation, stroke, dermatological complications and mood dysfunction have been described in the literature [6].

The Covid-19 pandemic radically altered people's lifestyles and had a major impact on public behaviour [7,8]. It has also led to a disruption in routine vaccination activities [9]. Vaccination against Covid-19 remains an essential means of controlling this pandemic. Phase 3 randomised controlled trials of different Covid-19 vaccines have shown efficacy rates ranging from 50% to 95%. Based on these results, the WHO and other health organisations have authorised the use of these vaccines from December 2020 [2].

Following this authorisation, the COVAX initiative was created to facilitate equitable access to vaccines for developing countries. This initiative is co-led by the Global Alliance for Vaccines and Immunization (GAVI) and its regular partners (WHO and UNICEF) with the Coalition for Epidemic Preparedness Innovations (CEPI) to accelerate the availability of vaccines at all levels [10].

The contagious and deadly nature of the Covid-19 pandemic called for a vaccine, and for the first time in history new technologies were used to develop vaccines, such as the mRNA vaccine and the adenovirus vaccine. The use of these new technologies was necessary to protect the world's population. This new technology has raised many public concerns about the imposition of an "experimental and untested" vaccine. In the news as enormous as Covid-19 requires the meticulous development of a new manual on the deployment and introduction of these vaccines in the context of a pandemic [11]. Initially, vaccination programmes were asked to exclude pregnant and breastfeeding women as priority targets, as clinical trial data at the time did not prove that the vaccine was safe for mothers and foetuses [12]. Countries will need to develop their plans taking into account the guidance provided by the WHO through COVAX. The aim of the National Covid-19 Vaccine Deployment Plan (NVDP) under the Expanded Programme on Immunisation (EPI) is to reduce morbidity and mortality due to this pandemic [13]. However, several countries offer these vaccines outside the EPI [2].

Senegal recorded its first case of Covid-19 on 02 March 2020. By 31 January 2021, all 14 regions had been affected and 77 of the 79 districts (97%) already had confirmed cases of Covid-19 [14]. In January 2021, the Comité Consultatif pour les Vaccins au Sénégal (CCVS) met to validate vaccination in the EPI:

• high morbidity and mortality, with 2,5127 confirmed cases and 592 deaths in January 2021,

• the existence of different safe and effective vaccines,

• the country's capacity to introduce new vaccines [15].

As part of its response to Covid-19, the country has drawn up a plan for the deployment of Covid-19 vaccines. Thanks to the vaccines acquired through bilateral cooperation and the COVAX initiative, the country was able to start vaccinating priority targets nationwide on 23 February 2021 through the usual EPI vaccination services. The general objective of this plan was to contribute to the reduction of morbidity and mortality linked to Covid-19 by vaccinating priority target populations. More specifically, this involved :

• vaccinate at least 90% of the priority target group (front-line healthcare workers, people aged 60 and over, people with chronic diseases) before June 2021;
• notify and manage 100% of cases of adverse events following vaccination (AEFI) recorded within 45 days of vaccination [14].

An intra-action review (IAR) was organised after 4 months of vaccination implementation. Its specific objectives were: (i) to analyse collectively the process and results of the Covid-19 vaccination response; (ii) to identify best practices and challenges in the implementation of Covid-19 vaccination; (iii) to improve the vaccination response by supporting best practices that contribute to achieving the programme's objectives and by taking steps to avoid gaps in the programme; (iv) generate recommendations and action points to improve implementation in subsequent phases; (v) document, share and apply lessons learned from response efforts for the benefit of overall health system strengthening [16]. In addition, the WHO recommends a post-introduction evaluation 6 to 18 months after the initial introduction of a Covid-19 vaccine, to answer questions about implementation performance and to guide future vaccination policy and strategies [17,18].

As of 30 February 2023, to our knowledge, no evaluation has been carried out since the introduction of COVID-19 vaccines into the EPI in Senegal. This is why we are conducting this study, which will enable us to: (i) identify the adjustments needed to the national vaccine deployment plan; (ii) optimise the management and use of Covid-19 vaccines; and (iii) provide lessons learned for future vaccine deployments in the event of a pandemic.The general aim of this study is to assess the preparation and implementation of the Covid-19 vaccination in Senegal's vaccination programme.

1.1 research

The main question of this study was: what was the quality of the programmatic aspects in the implementation of the PNDV and at all levels of the health pyramid? These areas were: regulatory; vaccine introduction planning and coordination; resources and financing; target populations and vaccination strategies; supply chain management and healthcare waste management; human resources management and training; vaccine acceptance and use; surveillance of adverse events following vaccination; vaccination monitoring system; disease surveillance; and evaluation of the introduction of Covid-19 vaccines.

1.2 Hypothesis

The deployment of Covid-19 vaccines in times of emergency is thought to be the reason why the indicators for the various programmatic aspects of the national vaccine deployment plan have not been achieved.

1.3 Objectives

General: Evaluate the preparation and implementation of the national plan for the deployment of Covid-19 vaccines in Senegal's vaccination programme.

Specific :

- analyse the implementation process ;

- measure the extent to which the indicators for implementing the deployment plan have been achieved

vaccines ;

- identify the obstacles or factors limiting the achievement of the indicators for the implementation of the vaccine deployment plan.

2 REVIEW OF LITERATURE

2.1 Definition of concepts

The origins of vaccination date back to the 7th century AD, when Indian Buddhists drank snake venom to "immunise" themselves against the effects of this toxin. But variolisation, the mother of vaccination, dates back to 16th century China. It consisted of administering a piece of cotton with pus from human pustules, which was then placed in the nostrils of an uncontaminated person, or using scales instead of pus, or having a healthy person wear the clothes of a sick person. Variolisation was first used in sixteenth-century India. In 1774, thanks to Benjamin Jesty, an Englishman, vaccination was achieved for the first time, after he noticed that milkmen seemed to be protected against smallpox after contracting vaccinia (cowpox). Between 1870 and 1885, with the efforts of Louis Pasteur and his students, modern vaccination and the first vaccines were developed [17]. The development of vaccination is summarised in the figure below.

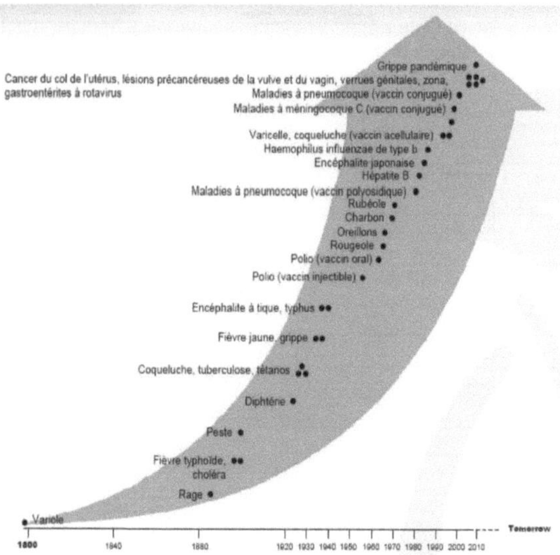

Figure 1: History of vaccination (Source: History and principles of vaccination.2019)

Expanded Programme on Immunisation (EPI): this is a government body responsible for immunisation. It was set up in response to a joint WHO/UNICEF report on high mortality from vaccine-preventable infectious diseases, which were one of the 5 leading causes of death in children under 5 in 1977 [19,20].

Vaccination: this is the artificial inoculation of an antigen into the body in order to induce an immune response. individual and collective immune response [18,21,22].

Vaccines: biological preparations, derived from the constituents or products of complete bacteria or viruses, whose capacity to produce the disease is reduced or removed by various processes, while retaining the capacity to induce a protective immune response. This makes them capable of preventing the onset of the disease or attenuating its clinical manifestations [21].

There are vaccines for both human and animal use. In this work, we will discuss the characteristics of vaccines for human use only. The different types of vaccine are summarised in the table below.

Table I: Classification of human vaccines by type

Type of vaccine	Definitions	Target diseases
Live attenuated vaccines	These are vaccines made from a pathogen that has been weakened.	Tuberculosis, smallpox, yellow fever, oral polio, measles, mumps, rubella, chickenpox, shingles, influenza, rotavirus, dengue fever, Japanese encephalitis, Ebola, Covid-19.
Inert vaccines	These vaccines are	Hepatitis A, injectable poliomyelitis, influenza
	completely	(fractionated), rabies, tick-borne encephalitis,
	without power	Japanese encephalitis, leptospirosis, cholera,
	infectious diseases, we have	tetanus, diphtheria, acellular pertussis,
	whole germ and	meningococcus B, hepatitis B, papillomavirus,
	sub-units.	pneumococcus (23 valences), typhoid,
		meningococcus AC and ACYW135,
		pneumococcus (13 valences), meningococcus C
		and ACYW135, Haemophilus influenzae type b,
		Covid-19

Most inert vaccines are combined with adjuvants. With the advent of Covid-19, in addition to the traditional attenuated and inert vaccines, there are also those based on DNA and ribonucleic acid (RNA). The RNA-based vaccine was developed by Moderna Therapeutics and Inovio Pharmaceuticals' and MERS, (Plymouth Meeting, PA, USA) on a new DNA vaccine [23,24].

Adjuvant: is a substance that enhances the immunity induced against the vaccine antigen with to which it is combined, by acting on the innate immune response [21].

COVAX: is the result of an extraordinary and unique global collaboration, with more than two-thirds of the world's population involved, it benefits from the largest and most diversified portfolio of vaccines against COVID-19 in the world. With the collaboration of the Accelerator, they aim to accelerate the development, production and equitable access to tests, treatments and vaccines against COVID-19 to end the acute phase of the disease at pandemic [25].

Following the approval of vaccines against Covid-19, several vaccines have been made available to countries, including [26].

BNT162b2 (COMIRNATY®): is a messenger RNA vaccine developed by Pfizer and BioNTech. It is administered intramuscularly in two doses, with the WHO recommending a 21-28 day interval between doses.

Comirnaty®: is a vaccine with 95% efficacy against symptomatic SARS-CoV-2 infection for use from the age of 6 months. Booster doses for children aged 5 to 11 and people aged 16 and over.

ChAdOx1 nCoV-19 (AZD1222, Vaxzevria®): is a vaccine developed in collaboration between Oxford University and AstraZeneca. It is 76% effective against symptomatic infection with SARSCoV-2. It is administered intramuscularly in two doses at an interval of 8 to 12 weeks.

Johnson & Johnson vaccine (Ad26.COV2-S, COVID-19 Vaccine Janssen): is a non-replicative viral vector vaccine effective in people with conditions associated with a higher risk of severe disease. It is administered as a single intramuscular dose. The WHO recommends a second booster dose for immunocompromised people aged 18 and over, in order to increase protection as quickly as possible.

mRNA-1273 (Spikevax®, COVID-19 Vaccine Moderna): is a messenger RNA vaccine co-developed by the Moderna laboratory and the NIAID vaccines, Spikevax®, which is 94.1% effective after the second dose.

BBIBP-Cor26: is a vaccine developed by Sinopharm that is administered in two doses by injection. intramuscular, at intervals of three to four weeks.

Sputnik V Sputnik V: is a non-replicative viral vector vaccine developed by the Russian institute Gamaleya. Its efficacy is 91.6% [26].

Health services system: the health services system is the set of actions designed to cover a range of specific health or social problems, from preventive to palliative services, including diagnostic and curative services. It includes the functions of public health care (surveillance, health protection and promotion, disease prevention, evaluation of health care delivery systems, development of public health skills), but not overall responsibility, affecting social, economic, cultural and demographic conditions [27]. The figure below shows the overall organisation of the healthcare system.

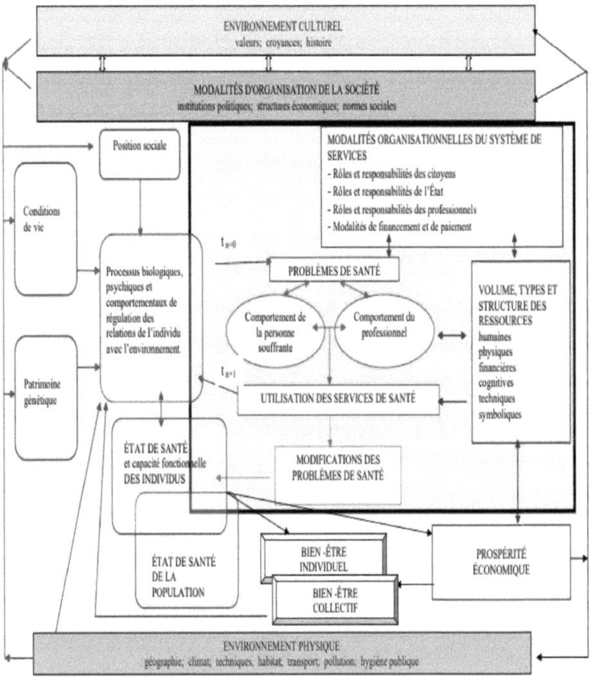

Figure 2: A global vision of the healthcare system (Source: EGIPSS. 2005)

Primary health care: primary health care is basic health care universally accessible to all individuals and families in a community by means acceptable to them, with their full participation and at a cost affordable to the community and the nation. Primary healthcare aims to combat the main health problems in the community and takes many forms: promotional, preventive, curative and rehabilitative actions [28].

Planning: is a dynamic process, whereby an organisation defines its objectives and the cycle is repeated at periodic intervals to take account of new developments [29]. See below for a schematic model of a strategic planning cycle.

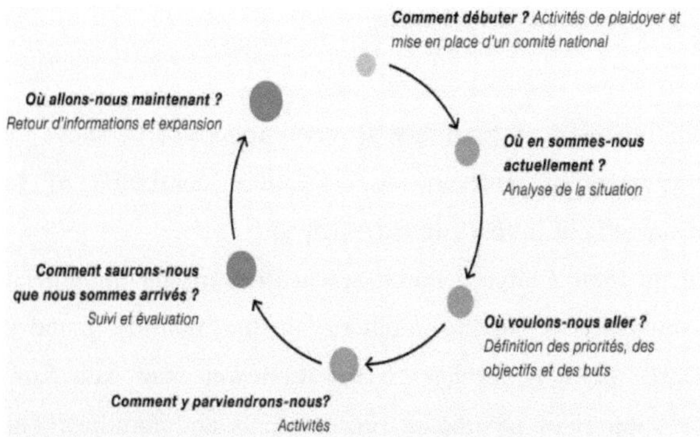

Figure 3: Schematic presentation of the planning and implementation cycle for a strategy (Source: WHO Manual for planning and monitoring national strategies)

Evaluation: a systematic and objective assessment of an ongoing or completed project or policy, its design, implementation and results. Its purpose is to determine the relevance and achievement of objectives, development efficiency, effectiveness, impact and sustainability [30]. The purposes of evaluation may be formal or informal. In this study, we will carry out a formal assessment as described in the table below.

Table II: Different purposes of programme/project evaluation

Strategic goal	Formative purpose	Summative purpose	Fundamental aim
Helping to plan and develop an intervention.	Providing information to improve an intervention along the way.	Determine the effects of an intervention in order to decide whether it should be maintained, substantially modified or discontinued.	Contribute to the advancement of knowledge and theoretical development.

In general, when new vaccines are introduced, these 4 aims (strategic, formative, summative and fundamental) are all used [31].

Performance of health service systems: the performance of health systems is defined according to several models, but according to the WHO, the performance of a health service system is the achievement of the best possible results from the system given the resources available [32].

2.2 Evaluation of vaccination programmes

Evaluation of immunisation programmes is very important to show the progress and challenges of implementing interventions, including continuity of service. Various studies have been carried out in this context, such as :

P. Gaudelus et al. in their study of the simplification of the immunisation schedule 2 years after its introduction among mothers on the internet found that data from immunisation records held by mothers were 3% lower than data from immunisation pages, despite the support of healthcare professionals and families. This suggests that communication with beneficiaries and healthcare professionals needs to be stepped up to ensure optimal coverage [33].

Similarly, a survey of vaccination coverage in Mayotte in 2010, carried out by J. Solet et al, showed that vaccination coverage was satisfactory for compulsory vaccines in children aged 2 to 4. However, it was inadequate for adolescents. This finding may be due, on the one hand, to the underestimation of vaccination coverage and, on the other hand, to the large number of vaccines used for this age group [34].

A study conducted by L. Sabiani on the evaluation of vaccination coverage for the human papillomavirus (HPV) vaccine in France from December 2009 to April 2010, with the aim of assessing the level of vaccination coverage of secondary school and university girls and their level of education about this vaccine, showed that only a minority of the target group had been vaccinated (35.4%). In addition to inadequate coverage, the vaccination schedule was not adhered to, thereby jeopardising the objective set by the introduction of the HPV vaccine [35].

In Côte d'Ivoire, in 2016, Yohou et al. reported inconsistencies between planning and implementation in their study on the "post introduction evaluation of the Haemophilus influenzae type b vaccine in the EPI". In fact, the introduction plan drawn up at central level was not disseminated to the regions and health districts [36]. Also in Côte d'Ivoire, Bénie Bi Vroh et al. in their study on the evaluation of the quality of immunisation data for children aged 0-11 months in 2012 revealed shortcomings in the accuracy of pentavalent vaccine data, showing that 23.3% of health districts overestimated vaccination unit data [37].

Another study conducted by M. Huré et al. in 2021 on the acceptability of the Sars CoV-2 vaccine in pregnant women showed that one of the factors associated with vaccination was advanced age, with a median age of 34 in the vaccinated population compared with 32 in the unvaccinated population. The vaccinated population also included a majority of managers (45.9%, 112/244), compared with a predominance of female employees in the non-vaccinated population (39.3%, 50/127) (p < 0,01) [38].

The study by T. Matuvanga et al. on the challenges to the introduction of the Covid-19 vaccine in the Democratic Republic of Congo in 2022 showed that the financial requests from the provinces were behind schedule, resulting in the non-implementation of planned activities. For example, the communication plan was never implemented. Failure to comply with the training plan led to missed opportunities, which were generally due to agents refusing to open vaccine vials if the target was not important [39].

In 2022, the Consultative Committee for Vaccination and Vaccines in Senegal (CCVS) carried out a study on the acceptability of vaccines against COVID-19 in Senegal. The study revealed a lack of reliable information on the usefulness and degree of efficacy of vaccines against COVID-19, which does not favour their acceptability. This low acceptability was also linked to insufficient information on side effects. An inequality in the transmission of information in favour of urban versus rural areas. In addition, vaccine stock-outs lead to missed opportunities [40].

In Senegal, the HPV vaccine was introduced nationwide in 2018 after a pilot phase in 9-year-old girls in three health districts (DS) (Dakar Ouest, Mékhé and Khombole). This study, carried out by Rebecca M. et al in 2022, reported that qualified staff were not permanently present at vaccination sites, leading to a mismatch in interpersonal communication and missed vaccination opportunities. In addition, despite the existence of a communication plan for the Human Papillomavirus (HPV) vaccine, stakeholders were confronted with information crises linked to rumours, which they were unable to resolve due to the lack of a crisis communication plan [41].

Following validation of the value framework by the WHO Strategic Advisory Group of Experts (SAGE) for the allocation of Covid-19 vaccines held on 26 August 2020, countries were guided on the allocation of Covid-19 vaccines and prioritisation of groups to be vaccinated [42].

The countries then drew up their national deployment and vaccination plans (NDPV) against Covid-19 in 2021. Senegal has taken the necessary steps to receive the first doses of vaccine from the first quarter of 2021 [43].

The WHO has provided countries with a checklist to facilitate a review of the successes of the process and the challenges in the first 6 months of Covid-19 vaccine deployment [43]. Post-vaccination evaluation is essential for any vaccine. Given that in the case of Covid-19, the vaccine was introduced under conditions of extreme urgency, there is a whole range of factors that contributed to vaccine hesitancy, such as inadequate information, the types of vaccine, the country of manufacture, equity, rumours, cultural and religious beliefs, etc., all of which could have affected the smooth introduction of the vaccine and public support for it. This assessment is therefore very important, as it is being carried out at a time when Covid-19 is no longer a public health emergency.

2.3 Administrative and territorial organisation of Senegal

Senegal has opted for a policy of administrative deconcentration, with 14 regions, 46 departments and 123 arrondissements. It is also implementing a policy of progressive and irreversible decentralisation, with 599 Collectivités Territoriales (CTs) (42 departments / CTs, 557 communes, including 3 towns, which follow the contours of their administrative department. Figure 1 shows Senegal's administrative regions [14].

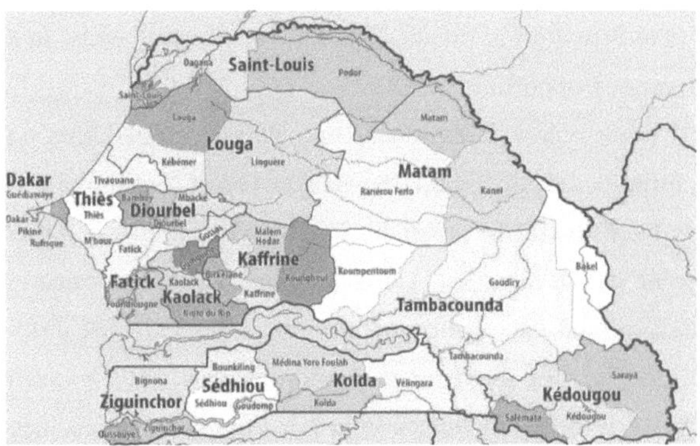

Figure 4: Administrative map of Senegal in 2023 (Source: PNDV)

2.4 Organisation of the health system in Senegal

Senegal's healthcare system is organised on a three-tier pyramid structure[45] :

☞ A **central level** comprising the Minister's Office, the General Secretariat, the Directorates-General, the National Directorates, the attached central departments, the National Social Reinsertion Centres and the level 3 Public Health Establishments;

☞ An **intermediate level** comprising the Medical Regions, the Regional Hygiene Brigades (BRH), the Regional Social Action Services (SRAS) and the level 2 Public Health Establishments;

☞ An **operational peripheral level** with Health Districts, Hygiene Sub-Brigades,

Departmental Social Action Services, Social Promotion and Reinsertion Centres (CPRS) and level 1 Public Health Establishments.

Figure 2 below shows the organisation of the Senegalese healthcare system.

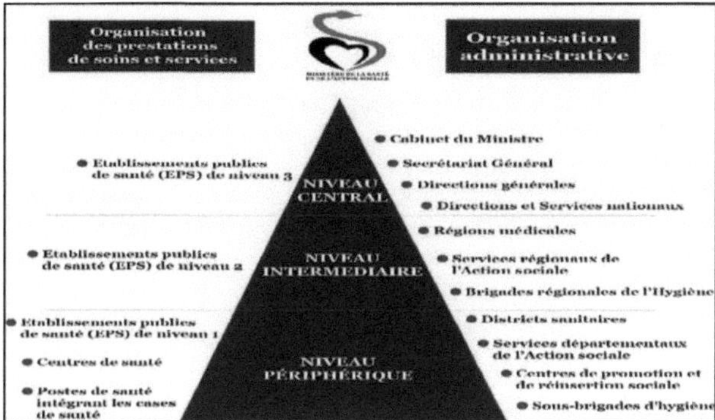

Figure 5: Organisation of the Senegalese healthcare system in 2023 (Source: PNDV)

2.5 Direction de la prevention

The Prevention Division comprises the Immunisation Division, the Prevention Division and the Prevention Division. epidemiological surveillance and vaccine response, which in turn is the responsibility of the Direction Générale de la Santé, the Division de la prévention individuelle et collective and the Programme national de lutte contre le tabac [45]. The following figure shows the organisation chart of the DP.

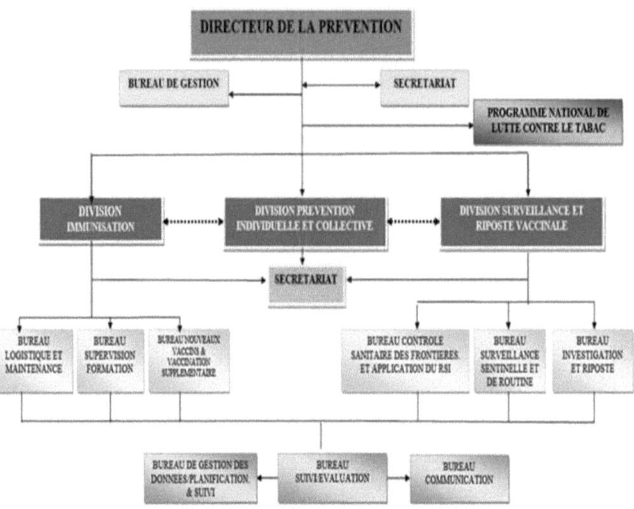

Figure 6: Organisation chart for the Prevention Department in 2023 (Source: report by situational analysis of vaccination)

2.5.1 History of the introduction of vaccines at Senegal

Senegal initiated the EPI in 1979, with the aim of reducing morbidity and mortality from vaccine-preventable diseases. When it was launched in 2004, the EPI targeted 7 diseases (tuberculosis, poliomyelitis, diphtheria, tetanus, whooping cough, measles and yellow fever) in children under the age of 1 [45]. From 2004 to 2018, 7 other vaccines against the following diseases were gradually added (hepatitis B, Haemophilus influenzae b infections, pneumococcus, rubella and measles (bivalent), rotavirus diarrhoea, poliomyelitis with the inactivated vaccine and human papillomavirus infections) [46].

Through these vaccination services, the programme offers vaccines against vaccine-preventable diseases to children aged 0-23 months, adolescents aged 9 years and pregnant women. The current vaccination schedules are shown in the tables below [45].

Table III: Vaccination schedule in force for children aged 0 to 23 months and adolescents aged 9 years in Senegal in 2023 (Source: Guide gestion PEV-SE Sénégal version 2023)

VACCINES	TARGET DISEASES	AGES
HEPB ZERO	Hepatitis b	Within 24 hours of birth
BCG	Tuberculosis	From birth to 3 months
VPO ZERO	Polio	From birth to day 14
PENTA1,VPO1, PCV13-1,ROTA-1, VPI 1	Diphtheria, tetanus, whooping cough, hepatitis b, Haemophilus influenzae type b infections, poliomyelitis Pneumococcal infections, rotavirus diarrhoea	6 weeks
PENTA2,VPO2, PCV13-2, ROTA-2		10 weeks
PENTA3,VPO3, PCV13-3, ROTA-3, VPI 2		14 weeks
RR1	Measles, rubella	9 months
VAA	Yellow fever	9 months
RR2	Measles, rubella	From 15 months
HPV	Papillomavirus infection human	From age 9

Table IV: Vaccination schedule in force for pregnant women in Senegal in 2023 (Source: Guide gestion PEV-SE Sénégal version 2023)

DOSES	TO ADMINISTER	LEVEL OF PROTECTION	DURATION OF PROTECTION
TD*1	On first contact with a woman of childbearing age; or as early as possible in pregnancy	None	No
TD2	At least 4 weeks after Td1	80%	3 years
TD3	At least 6 months after Td2	95%	5 years
TD4	At least 1 year after Td3	99%	10 years
TD5	At least 1 year after Td4	99%	For life

*TD = Tetanus Diphtheria

2.5.2 Performance of PEV

Since 2017, Senegal has seen a steady increase in administrative measles/rubella vaccine coverage for the first dose, from 70% to 85%, while the Demographic and Health Surveys (DHS) show a gradual decline from 88% to 61.5%. With regard to Penta-3, WHO/UNICEF estimates are superimposable on administrative data for 2017 and 2020. The reach every child (ACE) approach has been rolled out to all districts to improve immunisation coverage [45].

When analysing healthcare delivery systems, questions often relate to performance, efficiency, effectiveness, output, productivity, quality, access, equity and other concepts [27]. As performance is difficult to define, we have considered it here as the achievement of the objectives set by the EPI. The following table shows vaccination coverage according to administrative sources, DHS and WHO/UNICEF estimates for the national level from 2017 to 2021.

Table V: Vaccination coverage for BCG, Penta 1,3 and measles/rubella from 2017 to 2021 according to source (Administrative coverage, DHS and WUENIC).

YEAR	BCG			Penta 1			Penta3			RR1		
	Adm	EDS	WHO/UNICEF	Adm	EDS	WHO/UNICEF	Adm	EDS	WHO/UNICEF	Adm	EDS	WHO/UNICEF
2017	93	95	99	97	97	97	93	92	93	70	88	59
2018*	83	95	94	83	96	96	81	83	92	63	86	62
2019	103	94,5	95	106	96,2	97	100	92,1	95	78	61,5	68
2020	100		95	100		93	96		91	79		69
2021*	92		87	92		87	90		85	85		75

* 2018 was marked by a national strike by health workers (withholding of data and boycott of vaccination) which shows the higher coverage estimates than administrative ones. In 2021, we are seeing a drop in vaccination coverage, which could be linked to the onset of the Covid-19 pandemic.

3 METHODOLOGY

3.1 Type of study and period of study

This was a retrospective mixed-method cross-sectional evaluative study, from February to December 2021. Data collection took place from 02 to 14 July 2023 in the Dakar medical region (MR).

3.2 Framework

The study was carried out in the Dakar medical region. Dakar is the capital of Senegal, covering an area of 550 km2 with an estimated population of 4,146,621 in 2023, giving a population density of 7,349 inhabitants/km2. Administratively, it comprises 5 departments (Dakar, Pikine, Guédiawaye, Rufisque and Keur Massar) and 53 communes. According to the health division, it represents a medical region (intermediate level of the health pyramid). This medical region comprises 12 health districts (DS), 14 public health establishments (10 level 3, 1 level 2 and 3 level 1), 25 health centres (CS), 129 health posts (PS) and 39 health huts [39]. In addition to the public establishments, we have the private sector, as follows [47]:

- 65 clinics

- 218 doctors' surgeries

- 159 paramedical practices

- 16 health centres

- 20 health posts

- 1 Hospital

- 439 Pharmacies

- 141 Dental practices

- 52 Company Medical Services.

Below is the health map of the Dakar medical region.

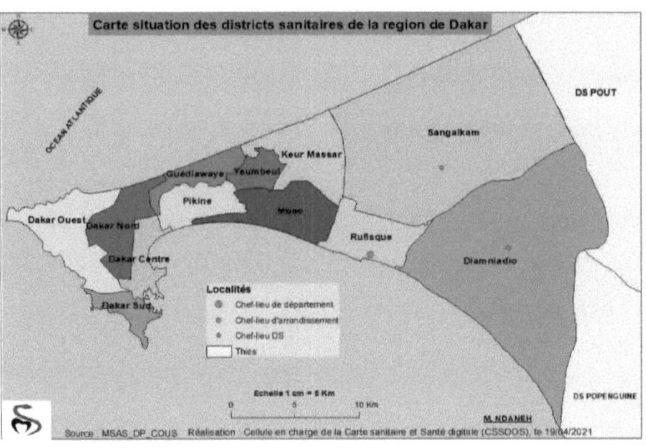

Figure 7: Health map of Dakar in 2021 (Source: MSAS).

The table below shows the population, surface area and density of the 5 departments in the Dakar medical region.

Table VI: Populations, areas and densities in 2021 of the districts in the Dakar medical region (Source: RM ACD plan).

Department	Health district	Population in 2021	Area in km2	Density inhabitants/km2
DAKAR	Dakar Centre	409384	13	29 350
	Dakar North	551188	22	23 034
	Dakar West	265951	34	7 281
	Dakar South	214894	10	20 390
GUEDIAWAYE	Guédiawaye	414519	13	29 536
KEUR MASSAR	Keur Massar	294157	34	7 957
PIKINE	Mbao	431266	28	14 114
	Pikine	413279	18	21 705
	Yeumbeul	333768	13	23 619
RUFISQUE	Diamniadio	163942	169	891
	Rufisque	278193	203	2 056
	Sangalkam	175886	195	902

3.3 Population study

It is made up of all the players involved in implementing the Covid-19 vaccine roll-out plan, at all levels of the health pyramid and meeting the selection criteria for this study. For the central level, the Prevention Directorate (DP) was chosen as the site and 5 people were interviewed: the Director of Prevention, the Head of the Immunisation Division, the Logistics Officer, the Communications Officer and the Head of the Surveillance Division;For the intermediate level, the Dakar medical region was chosen to take part in this survey, and 2 people were interviewed (the regional chief medical officer and the EPI focal point).For the peripheral level, the health districts (HDs) of Rufisque, Keur Massar and South Dakar were selected according to their performance (poor, average and good). In each health district, 3 people were surveyed (the head district doctor, the EPI focal point and the data manager). In addition to the health districts, 3 immunisation facilities were surveyed per health district and 3 people per facility: the head of the facility, the EPI agent and the data manager.

3.4 Inclusion criteria

All those involved in implementing the Covid-19 vaccination plan in the Dakar medical region and the prevention department were included in this study.

3.5 Sampling

To identify the sites and stakeholders for this study, we made a well-considered choice with reference to the WHO's Covid-19 vaccine post-introduction evaluation tool [2]. This choice enabled us to select sites involved in vaccination and people in charge of vaccination at all levels of the health pyramid, i.e. a total sample of 28 people to be interviewed.

3.6 Operational definition of the variables of interest

The variables in this study are taken from the different areas of the PNDV :

- **Regulatory preparedness**: regulation concerns marketing authorisation, emergency use and batch release through UNICEF's central purchasing office in Copenhagen. In emergencies or situations epidemic, a waiver of this release may be granted by the

Minister for Health. Cheers.

- **Planning and coordinating the introduction of the vaccine**: this area covers the following indicators (holding awareness-raising meetings with programme managers and chronic disease focal points, holding regular awareness-raising meetings with associations, holding regular meetings of regional/prefectoral coordination structures, holding meetings with the armed forces health service), to coordinate planning at all levels with all the parties involved.

- **Human and financial resources**: budgeting the costs of administering the vaccination against COVID-19.

- **Target populations and vaccination strategies**: mapping priority populations, identifying and analysing health interventions with a high potential for integrated delivery, taking into account the context and compatibility of interventions.

- **Supply chain management and cold chain management resulting from healthcare activities**: Strengthening vaccine storage and the cold chain, distribution planning and data management.

- **Acceptance and uptake of immunisation (demand)**: targeted strategies linked to demand and for more equitable access to quality services.

- **Vaccine safety monitoring, injection safety, management of MAPI and serious adverse events**: detecting any adverse events, whether expected or not, and dealing with them.

To measure the level of achievement of the indicators, we used three methods:

- **carried out**: meaning that the activity was fully implemented and sanctioned by a report or minutes ;

- **partially completed**: this is an activity that has been started but not yet completed, or that has been completed only partially.

breaking down the implementation stages ;

- **not carried out**: this refers to the failure to carry out a planned activity, whatever the reason.

For qualitative data we used the following terms:

- Strengths: these were their positive impressions of the activity.

- Areas for improvement: these were their negative feelings about the implementation of the activity.

And for the classification of districts we have defined performance as follows:

- Good performance was defined as vaccination coverage above the average for the medical region;

- average performance, with coverage equal to the average vaccination coverage in the medical region, and

- poor performance, with vaccination coverage below the average for the medical region.

Complete vaccination was defined as the receipt of a dose of Johnson & Johnson or 2 doses of any other vaccine.

3.7 Techniques and tools for collection

Data were collected using the WHO guide to the post-introduction evaluation of the Covid-19 vaccine (cPIE), 2021 edition, adapted to the country context. The Covid-19 Post-Introduction Evaluation (cPIE) tool is designed to provide a systematic method of evaluating a vaccination programme using structured interviews at national, sub-national and health facility levels, and with specific target groups in the community. It is also supplemented by systematic observations of vaccination sessions and vaccine storage sites. This tool is based on the publications "Post-introduction evaluation tool for new vaccines (PIE)1 and "Post-introduction evaluation of influenza vaccine "2 [48].

The objectives of a cPIE are as follows:

✓ highlight deployment activities that have gone well and should be maintained ;
✓ identify problems requiring corrective action ;
✓ highlight the lessons learned from the roll-out of the Covid-19 vaccine to strengthen the overall national immunisation system and services, particularly for health workers, the elderly, essential workers and people with co-morbidities;
✓ Make recommendations to improve the deployment of Covid-19 vaccines, particularly in terms of vaccinating progressive target groups and booster vaccination strategies;
✓ provide lessons learned from other countries for their own vaccine rollouts

against Covid-19 and for future deployment of vaccines in the event of a pandemic.

This form was entered into an Excel file, which was used as a data collection tool.

3.8 Sources of data

The study was based on semi-directive individual interviews and on consultation of the following documents:

- Covid-19 vaccine deployment plan, Covid-19 vaccination guidelines on vaccine products;
- the microplan (MR, DS and vaccination unit) ;
- activity reports (training report, database, minutes of meetings, supervision report, posters or leaflets, vaccination report; MAPI management directive, MAPI declaration form);
- Semi-structured individual interviews were conducted with those involved in formulating and/or implementing the Covid-19 vaccine deployment plan at all levels of the health pyramid (central, regional, district and health unit).

3.9 Processing and analysis of data

The data collected was entered into an Excel data mask and cleaned up by deleting duplicates, outliers and missing data. The database was then imported into Epi Info 7.2.5.0 for analysis, which enabled us to calculate frequencies for the various components of the PNDV. Qualitative data was collected according to the different areas of the plan, enabling us to complete the aspects not covered by the quantitative data. These data were collected at all the sites. At each level, the person in charge was interviewed alone about planning, coordination and finance. The technical staff (EPI focal point, communication and monitoring) were interviewed in focus groups. The interview focused on strengths, areas for improvement and lessons learned for each indicator.

3.10 Ethical considerations

For data collection, prior contact was made with all managers before the start of the fieldwork. The structures visited were informed two weeks in advance so that they could give us their consent and prepare the documentation.

4 RESULTS

A total of 13 sites involved in vaccination against Covid-19 were visited and the questionnaire was administered to 28 people. One site was excluded due to the unavailability of staff. The sites visited were

- Prevention Department ;

- Dakar Medical Region,

- three Health Districts;

- eight vaccination units.

4.1 Summary of the main indicators at the time of the post-introduction assessment anti-Covid-19 vaccines for all sites (n=13)

The evaluation grid is structured by domain, which enabled us to see all of the EPI components.In table VII, we have extracted certain relevant indicators for vaccine deployment to determine the level of implementation of NDPV activities. The indicators used in this table concern all the levels assessed in all the sites.

Table VII: Summary of the main NDPV indicators for all sites visited.

Main indicators	% directed	partly directed	%no directed
Awareness-raising meetings with programme managers and chronic disease focal points	38	0	62
Regular steering committee meetings held at least once a month	54	0	46
Update of microplans for the roll-out of vaccination against covid-19 by level	46	31	23
Carrying out routine covid-19 vaccination activities using existing EPI platforms	85	15	0
Vaccination training against covid-19	0	100	0
Organisation of local social mobilisation activities specific to the covid-19 vaccine	62	0	38
Existence of Covid-19 information media (posters) at vaccination sites	38	38	23
Existence of a procedure for MAPIs	100	0	0
Notification of a MAPI for vaccination against covid-19 since the start of vaccination	0	58	42
All MAPIs covered free of charge for vaccination against covid-19	0	0	100
Average achievement	42	24	33

Of all the indicators, we found that only the existence of a procedure for MAPIs was 100% achieved, three indicators were above 50% achievement and three others below 50%. The average score was 42%.

4.2 regulations

Table VIII sets out all the indicators for preparation in terms of regulations taken into account in our study.

Table VIII: Indicators of regulatory preparedness

Indicators	% achieved	% partially achieved	%not achieved
Emergency use authorisation	100%	0%	0%
Ensuring the conditions for importing WHO-approved vaccines	100%	0%	0%
Have an Import Authorisation	100%	0%	0%
Guarantee the Approval Mechanism approval or Exceptional Exemption Mechanism	100%	0%	0%
Take specific measures to manage the Covid-19 vaccine	100%	0%	0%
Average achievement	100%	0%	0%

All of the indicators for the regulatory preparation area were 100% compliant. These indicators only concerned the central level, which was represented by the Prevention Department with the support of the central pharmacy.

4.3 Planning and coordinating the rollout of Covid vaccines- 19

The NDPV planning and coordination indicators for the intermediate and peripheral levels are summarised in table IX below.

Table IX: Indicators for planning and coordinating the introduction of NDPV vaccines at the intermediate and peripheral levels.

Indicators	Region medical	District sanitary	Unit of vaccination
	(n= 1)	(n= 3)	(n= 8)
Awareness-raising meetings with programme managers and chronic disease focal points	100%	100%	13%
Regular meetings of technical groups	100%	0%	62%
Awareness-raising meetings with professional associations	100%	100%	63%
Update of microplans for the roll-out of vaccination against covid-19 in the Health Centres	100%	67%	25%
Average achievement	100%	63%	46%

For all the key NDPV planning and coordination indicators, we noted good performance (100%) for all the indicators at regional level. At the level of the health districts, the average achievement of all the indicators is 63%, and among these indicators we have the regular holding of meetings of the technical groups, which was not achieved by any health district. Similarly, only 25% of immunisation units updated their micro plans. Awareness-raising with programme managers and chronic disease focal points only reached 13% (1/8) of immunisation units.

4.4 Target populations and vaccination strategies

The table below shows the indicators relating to vaccination strategies.

Table X: Indicators on target populations and vaccination strategies.

Indicators	Region medical	District sanitary	Unit of vaccination
	(n=1)	(n= 3)	health (n=8)
Carrying out routine covid-19 vaccination activities using existing EPI platforms	100%	67%	88%
Vaccination training against covid-19	100%	100%	88%
Average achievement	100%	84%	88%

At this level, all the indicators remain acceptable, and the medical region has achieved 100% of all the indicators. At the level of the health districts, we note that 67% of the activities relating to the integration of existing platforms for the implementation of the PNVD have been carried out. Vaccination units achieved 88% of these indicators.

4.5 Supply and cold chain management

Table XI below provides information on the management of the cold chain and supply.

Table XI: Indicators on supply and cold chain management for the intermediate and peripheral level NDPV.

Indicators	Region medical	District sanitary	Unit of vaccination
	(n=1)	(n=3)	(n= 8)
Notification of cold chain problems	100%	67%	25%
Notification of stock-outs of covid-19 vaccine at the start of introduction	100%	100%	100%
Availability of several vaccine products against covid-19	100%	100%	100%
Average achievement	100%	89%	75%

For this area, all levels of the health pyramid had at least two vaccine products. Three quarters of immunisation units had at least one cold chain problem at the start of vaccine deployment. The medical region and the health districts reported cold chain problems of 100% and 67% respectively.

4.6 Acceptance and adoption of vaccination

Table XII below shows how communication took place at the following levels intermediate and peripheral.

Table XII: Indicator of acceptance and uptake of NDPV vaccination at the intermediate and peripheral levels.

Indicators				Medical region (n=1)	Health district (n=3)	Vaccination unit (n=8)
Organisation	Of activities	local	from	100%	100%	38%
social mobilisation specific to the covid-19 vaccine						
Existence of posters at vaccination sites				100%	100%	0%
Average achievement				100%	100%	19%

None of the health centres visited had posters on Covid-19 vaccination at their level and only 38% were carrying out social mobilisation activities. On the other hand, the medical region and the health districts had their communication plans and information posters on Covid-19.

4.7 Monitoring vaccine safety, managing MAPI and serious adverse reactions

The fundamental basis of prevention and control is surveillance, and the table below summarises the status of PNDV indicators in Senegal.

Table XIII: Vaccine safety monitoring indicators, management of intermediate and peripheral level NDPV MAPIs.

Indicators	Region medical	District sanitary	Unit of vaccination
	(n=1)	(n= 3)	(n=8)
Existence of a procedure for MAPIs	100%	100%	88%
Notification of at least one MAPI for the vaccination against covid-19 since the start of vaccination	0%	100%	63%
Free support for all MAPIs for vaccination against covid-19	0%	0%	0%
Total realisation	33%	67%	50%

With the exception of the existence of an IPD procedure, which is 100% at the level of the medical region and the health districts, the other indicators in this area are not appreciable. The medical region has not received any notifications of cases of MAPI from the districts, whether minor or major. The health districts and immunisation units that notified at least one case of IMD did not manage any cases either.

4.8 Analysis of qualitative data from interviews with healthcare professionals

The interview focused on strengths, areas for improvement and lessons learned for each indicator. It should be noted that 47% of respondents had nothing to say about these aspects. We therefore took into account the ideas that were mentioned most by the respondents, which we have summarised in the table below.

Table XIV: Main qualitative information obtained from interviews w i t h healthcare professionals on the 13 sites included, by domain.

Highlights	Areas for improvement
Planning and coordination of vaccine introduction	
Regular consultation with CNGE, CCVS, DGP. Purchase of the first doses by the State (200,000 doses), which enabled vaccination before the COVAX roll-out. Existence of EPI/ES focal points in each district. Existence of association platforms of healthcare professionals. Multi-sectoral approach to raising awareness among target groups. Support from the army for vaccinating priority targets. Involvement of community workers Involvement of local elected representatives in raising awareness.	No technical group meetings held at DS level. Delay in setting up funds for covid-19 vaccination. No meeting at the start of covid-19 at any level. High workload for the team DS managers and vaccinators.
Financial resources	
Collaboration between the players involved (office of the Minister of Health, Directorate of General Administration and Equipment, DP, Directorate of Disease Control, Child Survival, RM and DS) for 2 weeks to cost estimates. Existence of a decree to simplify disbursement procedures. Setting up a "covid-19 force" to implementation of covid-19 activities. Technical and financial support from international partners. Involvement of CDSs in the implementation of NDPV activities.	Administrative delays in disbursement, which took an average of 2 weeks. No line for "motivation "community health workers.

Highlights	Areas for improvement
Target populations and vaccination strategies	
Use of the same human resources for vaccination. Existence of an online platform for identifying elderly people living with co-morbidities. Integration of covid-19 activities into the DS's ACD plan.	Failure to take account of support staff when identifying the priority target (health workers). On-the-job training of health workers for the introduction of covid-19 vaccines (absence of hard copy and checklists). Age fraud (people claiming to be 60 or over) to obtain vaccination. Withholding of information on Covid-19 data at central level, for fear of revolt.
Ensuring supply chain management and cold chain management resulting from care activities	
Coinciding with the CCEOP1, making it easier to replace cold chains that have broken down. Existence of a waste collection plan at all levels.	Expiry dates close to those of the vaccines deployed. Vaccine failure at the start of vaccination at all levels. New shift managers are not familiar with the vaccine ordering tool (Logistimo).
Acceptance and adoption of vaccination (request)	
Existence of a RM rumours. Covid-19 sufferers testifying in the media (television), to confirm the existence of the disease and the need for a cure the importance of getting vaccinated.	Representatives not involved in drawing up the communication plan at local authority level. Lack of leaflets for interpersonal communication.
Monitor vaccine safety, manage MAPIs and effects serious unwanted	
Use of the same notification system as for other antigens. Existence of MAPI notification sheets.	Low notification of cases of MAPI Beneficiaries pay for MAPI.

4.9 Lessons

The Covid-19 pandemic was an unprecedented global experience that left many important lessons to be learned around the world. In the case of Senegal, we have the lessons below:

- motivate community players by involving them in other paid activities,

- existence of an electronic register to identify the priority target.

- purchase of the first doses by the state,

- existence of a derogation law to facilitate the disbursement of funds at the level of
the General Administration and Equipment Department,

- use of the usual EPI sites for vaccination against Covid-19,

- door-to-door vaccination campaigns for bed-ridden patients,

- redeployment of a working refrigerator from a low-target area to a high-target area with a
broken refrigerator,

- raising community awareness of antigen substitution.

5 ANALYSIS AND DISCUSSIONS

The roll-out of the Covid-19 vaccines took place in a special context. It has been 30 months since the introduction of this vaccine in Senegal, but no evaluation has been carried out. This was the reason for our study, the main objective of which was to assess the deployment of Covid-19 vaccines in the routine EPI in Senegal, in order to answer questions about the performance of this deployment, and to guide future vaccination policy and strategies.It is important to remember that Senegal was one of the first countries to introduce Covid-19 vaccines into the routine EPI before the WHO guidelines. This introduction was preceded by an intra-action review, the objectives of which were to document the lessons learned and generate action points for immediate implementation when preparing the subsequent phases of vaccine deployment. A post-deployment evaluation of the Covid-19 vaccines after two years was necessary to measure the level of achievement of the NDPV indicators. In this study we evaluated the first NDPV, which runs from February 2021 to December 2022, with the development of a recovery plan in August 2022.

5.1   regulations

This area concerned only the central level, and was 100% completed (Tab. VIII). This could be explained by the fact that in Senegal the (CCVS) is functional and dynamic. Moreover, the As soon as the pandemic was announced, the National Epidemic Management Committee (CNGE), set up in 2016, was reactivated. Its remit is to monitor trends in diseases with epidemic potential under surveillance; supervise the implementation of activities to prepare for, prevent and respond to all epidemics; and organise the evaluation of the response to epidemics.The CCVS sat in January 2021 for a systematic review on the criteria of immunogenicity, safety, tolerance, efficacy, conservation and storage using a planning tool (Logistic Planning Tool), cost and approval by international and national regulatory authorities [15]. This review enabled the CCVS to give its opinion on the deployment of Covid-19 vaccines in the country. It recommended a survey of the acceptability of vaccination against Covid19 as soon as possible, so that an evidence-based communication and training plan could be drawn up and implemented. M. Donadel et al in their systematic review, 2010-2020 on national decision-making for the introduction of new vaccines, highlighted that country ownership of immunisation programmes is a facilitator in the development of vaccine introduction policies [49].

Similarly, N. Ngcoba and N. Cameron have shown that the existence of a National Advisory Group on Immunisation (NAGI or NAGEI) has enabled the introduction of successful new vaccines in all countries, particularly developing countries, in their study of the decision-making process for the introduction of new vaccines in South Africa [50].

5.2 Planning and coordination of the introduction of vaccine

The main function of health planning is the management of health systems. It is considered to be a major event for health managers and technicians, and one which requires a great deal of time and resources. But these days, we see the influence of many partners in the process of drawing up national plans, making efficiency questionable. These documents are developed at great expense, with little follow-up [27].

The evaluation of the implementation of the planning and coordination of the introduction of the Covid-19 vaccines in the MR, the HDs and the immunisation units revealed different scores ranging from 50% for the HDs to 100% for the MR. This result corroborates that of Yohou et al. in 2016, in their study on the "post introduction evaluation of the Haemophilus influenzae type b vaccine in the EPI", who showed that the planning and coordination of this introduction had been carried out without any problems at 67% at regional level, 100% at district level and 92% at health facility level [36]. The low rate of planning and coordination observed at district level in our study was due to the fact that no meetings of technical groups were held, because of the heavy workload associated with the pandemic. Awareness-raising meetings with programme managers and chronic disease focal points at vaccination sites (13%) were only held in hospitals. The remainder was managed by the incumbent DS. It is important to note that the success of an introduction depended heavily on its micro-planning at operational level, i.e. at immunisation unit level. This micro-planning was only carried out by 25% of the sites, because of its emergency nature (barrier measures, distancing, etc.).

5.3 Target populations and vaccination strategies

Results in this area were generally satisfactory, ranging from 67% at the health district level to 100% at the regional level. Vaccination against Covid-19 was integrated into the routine EPI at all levels of the health pyramid at the same time. Unlike in the Democratic Republic of Congo, this was done gradually, starting with the most affected provinces on the basis of disease rates, the risk of spread and the willingness to distribute vaccines[51].

Senegal used the same routine vaccination staff for the Covid-19 vaccination as soon as the first doses of vaccine were available. And the guidelines for identifying targets were followed to the letter in all cases (100%) from the outset, even though managers were obliged to add support staff (guards, drivers, hygienists) to the list of health personnel. In addition, an electronic list was set up on a Ministry of Health and Social Action (MSAS) platform to identify elderly people (aged 55 and over) and those with co-morbidity(ies), designated as priorities for vaccination.However, vaccinators at the vaccination sites were trained on the job and without memory aids. This could be explained by the urgent integration of these vaccines at all levels. According to the WHO, failure to train vaccinators is one of the factors delaying vaccine deployment [43]. In Ghana and Côte d'Ivoire, for example, where training was carried out before the COVAX initiative vaccines were obtained, the deployment of COVID-19 vaccines was a success [13].

According to the health workers, the use of the same human resources has facilitated acceptance by the target population. This adherence should be materialised by good vaccination coverage, but the withholding of data (staff strike at peripheral level) did not allow us to make this observation.

5.4 Supply and cold chain management

The deployment of vaccines against Covid-19 coincided with the implementation of the cold chain optimisation platform (CCEOP) financed by GAVI [52]. This activity made it possible to strengthen the cold chain at the peripheral level, which explains the low level of notification. cold chain problems in only 25% of the immunisation units surveyed. However, these problems could have been even less frequent if the drafting of the national logistics plan for vaccination against covid-19 had not been delayed, with implementation 12 months after deployment. These results show that there were malfunctions in the cold chain at operational level. The regional and central levels did not report any difficulties related to the cold chain.The same applies to the Covid-19 vaccine stock-out at the start of the introduction, which was reported at all levels. These stock-outs could be explained firstly by a lack of control over the target (the priority population to be vaccinated) due to a lack of microplanning at grassroots level, and secondly by the vaccination of non-priority targets. According to Th. Baldé et al, in a study on the transition of the response to Covid-19 in the WHO African Region in 2022, Africa has been the victim of inequality in the deployment of vaccines, which has led to low vaccination coverage [53].

Browne et al, in their study on the evaluation of the new free family planning policy in Burkina Faso in 2022, found that the shortage of inputs was due to the high demand for services because of the free service. These shortages could be the cause of reluctance on the part of beneficiaries [54].

5.5 Acceptance and adoption of vaccination

Our study showed that the central, regional and district levels had drawn up communication plans for the deployment of Covid-19 vaccines. However, as we mentioned earlier, these plans did not take into account the specific characteristics of the vaccination sites. Social mobilisation was managed by all the HDs surveyed, but only 38% of immunisation units organised immunisation sessions in their localities with the support of the Health Development Committee (HDC), and no posters were found at the immunisation sites visited.Our results corroborate those of the 2016 study by S. Yohou et al, in Côte d'Ivoire, on the "post introduction evaluation of the Haemophilus influenzae type b vaccine in the EPI", which showed that no communication plan activities had been carried out at vaccination sites[36].Unlike the study by M. Waston et al in 2022 on the challenges of introducing the COVID-19 vaccine in the Democratic Republic of the Congo, the communication plan was not implemented at any level due to a lack of funding [55]. C. Wiysonge et al. in their study of vaccine hesitancy in the era of COVID-19 in 2021, suggested that before any new vaccine is introduced, the authorities should carry out anthropological studies to develop appropriate strategies to boost confidence in vaccination, since hesitancy may be vaccine-specific [56,57]. Issa. W, in his study on the challenges of efficiency in health systems planning in West Africa in 2018, tells us that in some countries such as Niger, despite a central planning system, health development plans are drawn up by local communities. This decentralisation makes it easier to monitor indicators on time [58].

5.6 Vaccine safety monitoring, injection safety, MAPI management and serious adverse events

Our study shows that there is an IPD management procedure at all levels of the health pyramid, even though in some vaccination sites we were unable to access the documents due to the redeployment of health staff. As far as notification of IPD is concerned, the RM informed us that in her zone, no cases of IPD had been notified, as only serious cases of IPD needed to be reported up the chain of command. The same applies to the districts and vaccination sites. On the other hand, at the peripheral level, we noted the existence of notification forms for minor IPD in all the health districts and in 63% of the vaccination sites. The few cases of IPD notified by health workers were managed by the beneficiaries. At the central level, we were able to verify that there were no funds for this purpose earmarked for the vaccination sites.

The multicentre study carried out in Burkina Faso and Mali by the CDC in 2012, on the evaluation of meningitis surveillance prior to the introduction of the serogroup A meningococcal conjugate vaccine, showed that despite the existence of procedures to monitor meningitis, cases notified at site level did not reach the central level for adequate decision-making [59]. Given that there has been an acceleration of results-based authorisation procedures, surveillance of MAPI remains the cornerstone of monitoring the safety of these vaccines [60]. In 2021, as part of the deployment of the Covid-19 vaccine in Africa, the WHO pointed out the inadequacy of many African countries in monitoring adverse events after vaccination [43].

6 LIMITS

Our study took place after the WHO declared the end of the Covid-19 pandemic emergency in May 2023 at the fifteenth meeting of the International Health Regulations (2005) Emergency Committee on Coronavirus Pandemic Disease 2019 [61]. This declaration reduced the use of services. In addition, front-line staff were withholding data, with the workers' union ordering staff not to release administrative data until they had won their case (pay rise). This withholding of data prevented us from comparing the coverage of the different sites visited. What's more, this evaluation, which was supposed to be carried out between 6 and 18 months after the introduction of vaccination anti-Covid-19 in the country, was only carried out in the context of our study after 30 months in a single region of Senegal, which is not representative of the whole country.

7 CONCLUSION

Post-introduction evaluation of Covid-19 vaccines is a WHO recommendation that enables Ministries of Health to highlight roll-out activities that have gone well and should be sustained, identify problems requiring corrective action, and highlight lessons learned from the roll-out of the Covid-19 vaccine to strengthen the overall national immunisation system and services. Our study showed that deployment of the Covid-19 vaccine did indeed take place at all levels of the health pyramid, using the same routine immunisation system.Nevertheless, some planned activities have not been implemented at all levels of the health pyramid such as:

- The meetings of the technical groups in the Health Districts have had an impact on the monitoring of activities at the vaccination sites, which could help to correct shortcomings;
- Social mobilisation activities for vaccination at vaccination sites can have several negative consequences on vaccination efforts and could be the reason for misinformation in our context;
- setting up communication media (posters) at vaccination units can leave targets without the information they need to make informed decisions about their health. These materials play a crucial role in providing essential information on prevention methods;
- the management of MAPI, which, if it is not effective, could create a bad perception of vaccines, with individuals hesitating to be vaccinated for fear of developing undesirable symptoms without adequate recourse.

These shortcomings mean that the roll-out of vaccines against Covid- 19 did not enable the indicators for the various programmatic aspects of the national vaccine deployment plan to be achieved.A nationwide study involving beneficiaries could further identify the advantages and disadvantages of deploying vaccines using our approach.

8   RECOMMENDATIONS

The evaluation of strategic plans is a systematic and objective assessment of a project. The WHO recommends a post-introduction evaluation 6 to 18 months after the initial introduction of a vaccine against Covid-19, to answer questions about the impact of the vaccine on the patient's health.performance to guide future policy and implementation strategies. vaccination [17,18]. At the end of our study, given all the findings, we suggest :
- the General Administration and Equipment Department: to make the funds available to the entities responsible for implementing the activities;
- the Prevention Department: for the roll-out of new vaccines, to hold specific meetings for close monitoring and to provide incentives for community civil servants. The same applies to the free treatment of MAPI.
- Health districts: to organise micro-planning workshops from the health centres/posts upwards to the health districts, involving community and religious leaders. And to organise training with the distribution of teaching materials;

- technical and financial partners: to avoid buying expiring vaccines close.

9 REFERENCES

1. Migliani R. La pandémie de Covid-19, spécificités en Afrique. Hérodote. 2021;183(4):85-97.

2. Patel MK, Bergeri I, Bresee JS, Cowling BJ, Crowcroft NS, Fahmy K, et al. Evaluation of post-introduction COVID-19 vaccine effectiveness: Summary of interim guidance of the World Health Organization. Vaccine. 5 Jul 2021;39(30):4013-24.

3. Eboko F, Schlimmer S. COVID-19: Africa faces a global crisis. Foreign Policy. 2020;Hiver(4):123-34.

4. WHO Coronavirus (COVID-19) Dashboard [Internet]. [cited 30 Dec 2022]. Available from: https://covid19.who.int

5. Sharif N, Alzahrani KJ, Ahmed SN, Dey SK. Efficacy, Immunogenicity and Safety of COVID-
19 Vaccines: A Systematic Review and Meta-Analysis. Front Immunol. 11 Oct 2021;12:714170.

6. Desai AD, Lavelle M, Boursiquot BC, Wan EY. Long-term complications of COVID-19. Am J Physiol Cell Physiol. 1 Jan 2022;322(1):C1-11.

7. Boespflug M, McLaughlin C, Pelletier P. Mieux connaitre les populations pour une communication de crise efficiente - Le cas de la pandémie de COVID-19.

8. Ibrahim NK. Epidemiologic surveillance for controlling Covid-19 pandemic: types, challenges and implications. Journal of Infection and Public Health. 1 Nov 2020;13(11):1630-8.

9. MacDonald NE, Comeau JL, Dubé È, Bucci LM. COVID-19 and missed routine immunizations: designing for effective catch-up in Canada. Can J Public Health. August 2020;111(4):469-72.

10. COVAX facility [Internet]. [cited 6 Sep 2023]. Available from: https://www.gavi.org/covax- facility

11. Poland GA. Tortoises, hares, and vaccines: A cautionary note for SARS-CoV-2 vaccine development. Vaccine. 2 June 2020;38(27):4219-20.

12. Zipursky JS, Greenberg RA, Maxwell C, Bogler T. Pregnancy, breastfeeding and the SARS-CoV-2 vaccine: an ethical framework for shared decision-making. CMAJ. May 17, 2021;193(20):E750-2.

13. Ghana shares success story in COVID-19 vaccine rollout with Cote d'Ivoire [Internet]. WHO Regional Office for Africa. 2023 [cited 14 August 2023]. Available from at: https://www.afro.who.int/news/ghana-shares-success-story-covid-19-vaccine-rollout- cote-divoire

14. Ministry of Health and Social Action. Plan de déploiement vaccin covid.docx [Internet]. Google Docs. 2021 [cited 12 March 2023]. Available from: https://docs.google.com/document/d/1DQ1hiIQ4pMlaZDYIFpEeNeesFxsrM7fa/edit?usp =drive_web&ouid=101069346929064625995&rtpof=true&usp=embed_facebook

15. Consultative Committee for Vaccination in Senegal (CCVS). CCVS recommendations for the introduction of a vaccine against the coronavirus (sars-cov2) responsible for covid-19 infection. 2021.

16. Prevention Department. REPORT OF THE INTRA-ACTION REVIEW (IAR) ON VACCINATION AGAINST COVID-1. 2021.

17. Canouï E, Launay O. History and principles of vaccination. Revue des Maladies Respiratoires. 1 Jan 2019;36(1):74-81.

18. Dupire G, Pijpen N, Elleni V, Michel O, Said BB. Efficacy of tolerance induction to COVID-19 Comirnaty Pfizer mRNA vaccine in a series of 7 cases of proven anaphylaxis to PEG or polysorbate. Annales de Dermatologie et de Vénéréologie-FMC. 2022;2(8):A60.

19. Mr Samou DEMBÉLÉ. Covid-19: the current state of routine childhood immunisation in France. commune V of the district of Bamako. 2022.

20. Santoni F. The Expanded Programme on Immunization: 25 years tomorrow.

21. UNICEF. Practical manual on immunization for health professionals [Internet]. 2015 [cited 14 March 2023]. Available from at: https://www.sante.gov.ma/Publications/Guides-Manuals/Documents/manual%20practice%20on%20the%20vaccination%202015%20.compressed.pdf

22. Espesson-Vergeat B, Morgon P. The challenge of vaccine prevention: overcoming personal rather than microbiological resistance. Droit, Santé et Société. 2019;3(3):47-64.

23. Pauline Maisonnasse, Frédéric Martinon. The long history of messenger RNA vaccines [Internet]. 2021 [cited 13 June 2023]. Available from: https://www.larecherche.fr/la-longue- histoire-des-vaccins-à-arn-messager

24. Gavriatopoulou M, Ntanasis-Stathopoulos I, Korompoki E, Fotiou D, Migkou M, Tzanninis IG, et al. Emerging treatment strategies for COVID-19 infection. Clin Exp Med. May 2021;21(2):167-79.

25. COVAX explained | Gavi, The Vaccine Alliance [Internet]. [cited 6 Sep 2023]. Available from: https://www.gavi.org/vaccineswork/covax-explained

26. Coronavirus disease 2019 (COVID-19): vaccines [Internet]. [cited 11 Sep 2023]. Available from:https://www.who.int/fr/news-room/questions-and-answers/item/coronavirus-disease-(covid-19)-vaccines

27. 200509_modeleEGIPSS.pdf [Internet]. [cited 1 Sep 2023]. Available from: https://www.csbe.gouv.qc.ca/fileadmin/www/Archives/ConseilSanteBienEtre/Rapports/200509_modeleEGIPSS.pdf

28. World Health Organisation. Alma Ata, primary health care. 1978.

29. World Health Organization. Manual for planning and monitoring national strategies for ear and hearing care [Internet]. World Health Organization; 2016 [cited 1 Sep 2023]. 39 p. Available from: https://apps.who.int/iris/handle/10665/208899

30. Austrian Development Cooperation. Guide to the evaluation of projects and programmes [Internet]. 2009 [cited 15 March 2023]. Available from: https://www.oecd.org/development/evaluation/dcdndep/47069377.pdf

31. Hartz (ed.) B Astrid, François Champagne, André Pierre Contandriopoulos and Zulmira. Evaluation: concepts and methods: second edition. Les Presses de l'Université de Montréal; 2011. 429 p.

32. World Health Organisation. Comparative analysis of health systems - The concept of health system performance: an example of an approach, the WHO study [Internet]. [cited 1 Sep 2023]. Available from: https://fad.univlorraine.fr/pluginfile.php/23862/mod_resource/content/1/co/Notion%20de%20performance%20des%20systemes%20de%20sante%20Un%20exemple%20dapproche%2C%20let ude%20de%20lOMS.html

33. Gaudelus J, Denis F, Cohen R, Stahl JP, Pujol P, Gauthier E, et al. Is the simplification of the vaccination calendar being applied? Assessment 2 years after its implementation. Archives de Pédiatrie. 1 Oct 2016;23(10):1012-7.

34. Bernier A, Goaster C, Pègue-Lafeuille H, Floret D. Survey on the delivery of immunoglobulin prophylaxis after exposure to a case of measles, France, 2010- 2011. Bulletin Epidemiologique Hebdomadaire. 19 Feb 2013;

35. L.Sabiani et al E. Évaluation de la couverture vaccinale du vaccin anti-hpv : résultats d'une enquête auprès des lycéennes et étudiantes de la région PACA [Internet]. EM-Consulte. 2011 [cited 20 March 2023]. Available from: https://www.em-consulte.com/article/703518/evaluation-de-la-couverture-vaccinale-du-vaccin-an

36. Yohou KS, Lépri-Aka N, Noufe S, Douba A, Assi Assi B, Dagnan NS. Evaluation of the introduction of haemophilus influenzae vaccine in Côte d'Ivoire. Santé Publique. 2016;28(5):655-64.

37. Bénie Bi Vroh J, Noufé S, Tiembre I, Bogui TY, Lepri NA, Yohou KS, et al. Quality of vaccination data in children aged 0-11 months in Côte d'Ivoire. Santé Publique. 2015;27(2):257-64.

38. Huré M, Peyronnet V, Sibiude J, Cazenave MG, Anselem O, Luton D, et al. Acceptability of the Sars CoV-2 vaccine in pregnant women, a cross-sectional questionnaire survey. Gynecologie, Obstetrique, Fertilite & Senologie. Nov 2022;50(11):712.

39. Zola Matuvanga T, Doshi RH, Muya A, Cikomola A, Milabyo A, Nasaka P, et al. Challenges to COVID-19 vaccine introduction in the Democratic Republic of the Congo - a commentary. Hum Vaccin Immunother. 30 Nov 2022;18(6):2127272.

40. Comité Consultatif pour la Vaccination au, la Vaccination au, Sénégal (CCVS). Acceptability of COVID-19 vaccines in Senegal. 2022 March.

41. Casey RM, Adrien N, Badiane O, Diallo A, Loko Roka J, Brennan T, et al. National introduction of HPV vaccination in Senegal-Successes, challenges, and lessons learned. Vaccine. 31 March 2022;40 Suppl 1:A10-6.

42. World Health Organization. WHO SAGE value framework for allocating COVID-19 vaccines and prioritizing groups for vaccination [Internet].2020 Sept. Available at: https://apps.who.int/iris/bitstream/handle/10665/336541/WHO-2019-nCoV-

SAGE_Framework-Allocation_and_prioritization-2020.1-
fre.pdf?sequence=1&isAllowed=y

43. World Health Organization. Risks and challenges in Africa's COVID-19 vaccine
rollout [Internet]. WHO | Regional Office for Africa. 2023 [cited 14 August 2023].
Available from: https://www.afro.who.int/news/risks-and-challenges-africas-covid-19-
vaccine- rollout

44. WHO C. National deployment and vaccination plan for COVID-19 [Internet]. 2021.
Available from: WHO reference number: WHO/2019-
nCoV/NDVP/country_plans/2021.1

45. Prevention Department. Comprehensive Multi-Annual Plan (cMYP 2019-2023). 2018.

46. Direction générale de la sante direction de la prévention. Guide de gestion du programme
élargi de vaccination et de la surveillance épidémiologique. 2023.

47. Dakar medical region. ACE PLAN OUTLINE. 2023.

48. World Health Organization O. Guidance for post-introduction evaluation of COVID-
19 vaccine (cPIE): provisional guidelines, 25 August 2021 [Internet]. World Health
Organization Health;2021. Available at:
https://apps.who.int/iris/bitstream/handle/10665/352126/WHO-2019-nCoV-cPIE- 2021.1-
eng.pdf

49. Donadel M, Panero MS, Ametewee L, Shefer AM. National decision-making for the
introduction of new vaccines: A systematic review, 2010-2020. Vaccine. 1 Apr
2021;39(14):1897-909.

50. Ngcobo NJ, Cameron NA. The decision making process on new vaccines introduction
in South Africa. Vaccine. 7 Sep 2012;30:C9-13.

51. Zola Matuvanga T, Doshi RH, Muya A, Cikomola A, Milabyo A, Nasaka P, et al.
Challenges to COVID-19 vaccine introduction in the Democratic Republic of the Congo -
a commentary. Human Vaccines & Immunotherapeutics. 30 Nov 2022;18(6):2127272.

52. Prevention Department. Plan national logistique de la vaccination contre la covid-19 au
Sénégal. 2022.

53. Balde T, Oyugi B, Byakika-Tusiime J, Ogundiran O, Kayita J, Banza FM, et al.

Transitioning the COVID-19 response in the WHO African region: a proposed framework for rethinking and rebuilding health systems. BMJ Glob Health. 29 Dec 2022;7(12):e010242.

54. Browne L, Cooper S, Tiendrebeogo C, Bicaba F, Bila A, Bicaba A, et al. Using experience to create evidence: a mixed methods process evaluation of the new free family planning policy in Burkina Faso. Reprod Health. 18 March 2022;19:67.

55. Watson M, Shaw D, Molchanoff L, McInnes C. Challenges, lessons learned and results following the implementation of a human papilloma virus school vaccination program in South Australia. Australian and New Zealand Journal of Public Health. 1 August 2009;33(4):365-70.

56. Wiysonge CS, Ndwandwe D, Ryan J, Jaca A, Batouré O, Anya BPM, et al. Vaccine hesitancy in the era of COVID-19: could lessons from the past help in divining the future? Hum Vaccin Immunother. 31 Dec 2022;18(1):1-3.

57. MacDonald NE. Vaccine hesitancy: Definition, scope and determinants. Vaccine. August 14, 2015;33(34):4161-4.

58. Wone I. The challenges of efficiency in health systems planning in West Africa. l'Ouest. Public Health. 2018;30(6):905-9.

59. Centers for Disease Control and Prevention (CDC). Evaluation of meningitis surveillance before introduction of serogroup a meningococcal conjugate vaccine - Burkina Faso and Mali. MMWR Morb Mortal Wkly Rep. 21 Dec 2012;61(50):1025-8.

60. Bertholom C. Covid-19 vaccines: where do we stand? Option/Bio. 2021;32(627):18-9.

61. Statements [Internet]. [cited 11 Sep 2023]. Available from: https://www.who.int/fr/news-room/statements

Appendix 1: addresses of people interviewed

First and last names	Function	mail address	Phone number
Rufisque Health District			
Dr Diabel DRAME	Chief Medical Officer DU DS	diabeldrame@yahoo.fr	+221 77 645 60 78
Ms Fatoumata Diakité	EPI and Surveillance Focal Point	fajules19744@gmail.com	+221 77 612 04 07
Mr Mamadou Sahir Diallo	Head nurse Diorga	msahirdiallo@gmail.com	+221 77 565 82 35
Mr Cheikhou Kanté	Community agent	chekhoukanté6@gmail.com	+221 77 659 39 91
Ms Seynabou Ndiaye	EPI focal point	naboundiaye86@gmail.com	+221 77 508 03 28
Ms Aissatou Diop	EPI focal point	massambacherif3@gmail.com	+221 77 847 28 92
Mrs Fawadou Wele Gaye	Station Manager Gouye	fawadeguaye@gmail.com	+221 77 464 62 37
Dakar South Health District			
Dr Maty DIOUF	Chief Medical Officer	sakhomaty@gmail.com	+221 77 645 60 78
Ms Aicha KEBE	DS EPI Focal Point	Achaamar2@gmail.com	+221 77 255 15 15
Ms Khary NDOYE	DS Communication Focal Point	tatoute2020@gmail.com	+22178 466 81 05
Mr Mailck SARR	Surveillance focal point	malicksarr65@gmail.com	+221 77 538 57 08
	epidemiology of DS		
Ms Fatou Ndoye	Head of the Health Centre		+221 77 378 77 52
Mrs Soukoura Diakhaté GUISSE	EPI Manager for the South Health Centre		+22177 439 96 94
Mrs MBOW	EPI Manager for Abass NDAO Hospital		+221 77 510 70 74

Mr Pape Ibrahima SALL	EPI manager for the Sandial Socialist Party		+221 77 366 72 58
MR BADJI	Head of PS Sandial		+221 78 160 16 69
Keur Massar health district			
Dr Amady BA	Chief Medical Officer	bamady1@yahoo.fr	+221 77 541 48 80
Mrs Fatma Ngoye Touré	DS EPI Focal Point	fatmangoyetoure@gmail.com	+221 77 542 34 61
Mr Babacar MBOUP	Head of PS Mrs Fatou Ba		
Mr Ousmane THIOMBA NE	Head ofPS Keur Massar village		
Medical region			
Dr Aly Ngoné TAMBEDOU	Doctor Head of the BRISE	tambedou_aly@yahoo.fr	+221 77 535 58 64
Ms Mame Diarra DIAGNE	RM EPI focal point	diaradiagne1@gmail.com	+221 77 490 56 59
Central level			
Dr Ousseynou Badiane	Head of Immunisation Division	ouzbad@hotmail.com	+221 77 651 43 76
Dr Boly DIOP	Head ofsurveillance division	diopboly@yahoo.fr	+221 77 531 99 63
Dr Abdoulaye MANGANE	Manager deputy immunisation	abdoulayemangane@yahoo.fr	+221 77 557 88 50
Dr Youssouf MBAYE	Immunisation	youmbaye9@yahoo.fr	+221 77 550 08 23
Dr Amy LO	Manager	amyndiayelo1@gmail.com	+221 77 566
	logistics		14 22

Domains	Labels	MOE status	Highlights	Areas for improvement
I. Regulatory readiness n (Documentation available, challenges, collaboration with pharmacy)	1 Emergency use authorisation			
	2.Ensuring the conditions of vaccine imports WHO-approved			
	3. Authorisation import			
	4 Guaranteeing the Mechanism approval or exemption exceptional			
	5.Taking specific measures for vaccine management against Covid-19			
II. Planning and coordination of the introduction of the vaccine (Pers. Resource for drawing up the plan,	6. ensure the regular maintenance of Steering Committee meetings			
	7. ensure the regular maintenance of Technical Committee meetings			
	8.ensure the regular maintenance of CCVS meetings			
	9. ensure regular meetings of regional coordination structures			
	10. hold regular structure meetings prefectoral coordination			
the impact of meetings)	11. update the Covid-19 vaccination roll-out microplans at local level regions			
III. Resources and financing the elements covered by the plan, activity limited by default of funding	12. draw up a budget estimate for the implementation of the PNDV			
	13.mobilise funding by source			

IV. Target populations and vaccination strategies (how the target groups were targeted and the strategies used)	14. name the priority targets			
	15. ensure routine vaccination activities against COVID-19 by integrating existing EPI platforms			
	16 Organize quarterly booster vaccinations or intensified vaccination (mass vaccination campaigns) to complement the vaccination of the population. routine			
	17. train health workers in vaccination against COVID-19			
V. Managing the supply chain and management of waste resulting from the company's activities care.	18. have a Covid-19 vaccination logistics plan that takes into account the various aspects of logistics			
	19. Quantification of vaccine and other input requirements			
	20. Management tools			
	21. Waste management			
VII. Guaranteeing Acceptance and Adoption of the vaccination (request)	22. draw up a communication			
	23 Production and distribution of information and promotional materials.			
VIII. Ensuring Monitoring	24. manage MAPIs at all levels			
vaccine safety, injection safety, management of MAPI and adverse reactions serious	25. Describe the procedure for MAPIs			
Summary	Total			
	Rate of completion			

Appendix 3: Questionnaire for the regional and district levels

Domains	Labels	Status of MEO	Points strong	Points to improve
I. Planning and coordination the introduction of the vaccine	1. Hold an awareness-raising meeting with the heads of programme and disease focal points chronicles			
	2. ensure regular meetings of the technical groups			
	3) Hold an awareness-raising meeting with professional associations (doctors/nurses/midwives, healthcare staff, etc.). companies, ASPS, etc.)			
	4. ensure regular meetings of regional/prefectoral coordination structures			
	5.meet with the health of the armed forces			
	6.update micro plans deployment of vaccination against Covid-19			
II. Resources and financing	7. carry out the activities implementation of Covid-19 vaccines in the EPI			
	8. name the priority targets			
III. Target populations and vaccination strategies	9. carry out routine vaccination activities against COVID-19 by integrating the existing platforms of the EPI			
	10) Organise quarterly booster vaccinations or intensified vaccination (mass vaccination campaigns) to complement routine vaccination.			
	11.90% of the target group vaccinated priority 2021			
	12.provide training for Health on vaccination against COVID-19			

IV. Managing the supply chain and management of waste resulting from healthcare activities.	13. ensure that COVID vaccines are included in orders periodic PPS and DS			
	a. List the establishments that have reported a cold chain capacity insufficient			
	b. Systematically draw up a monthly stock situation			
	c. Name the vaccination units that have observed or reported cold chain problems since the introduction of the new vaccine			
	e. Describe the challenges associated with delivery or collection vaccines tovaccination			
	cite the number of incinerators waste			
	several COVID-19 vaccine products are available			
V. Management and training	14. train and retrain health workers in anti-COVID vaccination			
human resources	15.carry out site supervision from the introduction of the COVID-19			
VI. Ensuring acceptance and adoption of the vaccination (request)	16. draw up a communication and social mobilisation plan specific to the vaccine against COVID-19			
	17.develop and disseminate messages tailored to the vulnerable persons			
VII. Monitoring the safety of vaccines, injection safety, MAPI management and adverse reactions serious	21. Notify 100% of cases of MAPI			
	22. Take charge of all MAPIs for vaccination against COVID-19			
Summary	Total			
	Rate of completion			

Appendix 4: Questionnaire for vaccination units

Domains	Labels	Status of MEO	Points strong	Points to improve
I. Planning and coordination the introduction of the vaccine	1. ensure the regular maintenance of technical group meetings			
	2) Hold an awareness-raising meeting with professional associations (doctors/nurses/midwives, healthcare staff, etc.). companies, ASPS, etc.)			
	3. update the micro plans for deploying vaccination against Covid-19 in the Health Centres			
II. Resources and funding	4. carry out the activities implementation of Covid-19 vaccines in the EPI			
III. Target populations and vaccination strategies	5. name the priority targets			
	6. ensure routine vaccination activities against COVID-19 by integrating existing EPI platforms			
	7) Organize quarterly booster vaccinations or intensified vaccination (mass vaccination campaigns) to complement the vaccination of the population.routine			
	8.90% of 2021 priority target vaccinated			
	9.train healthcare staff on vaccination against COVID-19			
IV. Managing the supply chain and management of waste resulting from healthcare activities.	10. ensure that COVID vaccines are included in orders periodic PPS and DS			
	a. List the establishments that have reported a cold chain capacity insufficient			

	b. Systematically draw up a monthly stock situation			
	c. Name the vaccination units that have observed or reported cold chain problems since the introduction of new vaccine			
	e. Describe the challenges associated with delivery or collection from vaccines to establishments/vaccination sites			
	f. Name the number of waste incinerators			
	g. arrange several products vaccines against COVID-19			
V. Managing and human resources training	11.train and retrain health workers on COVID vaccination			
	18.carry out site supervision from the introduction of the COVID-19			
VI. Ensuring acceptance and adoption of the vaccination (request)	19. draw up a communication and social mobilisation plan specific to the vaccine against COVID-19			
	20 Design and disseminate messages tailored to vulnerable groups			
VII. Monitoring the safety of vaccines, injection safety, MAPI management and adverse reactions serious	21. Notify 100% of cases of MAPI			
	22. Take charge of all MAPIs for vaccination against COVID-19			
	23. Describe the procedure for MAPIs			
Summary	Total			
	Rate of completion			

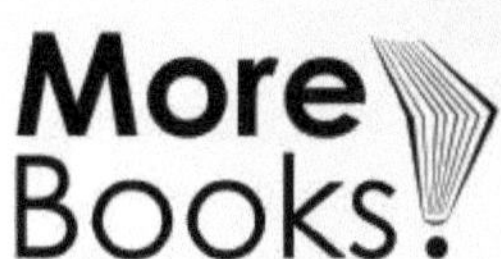

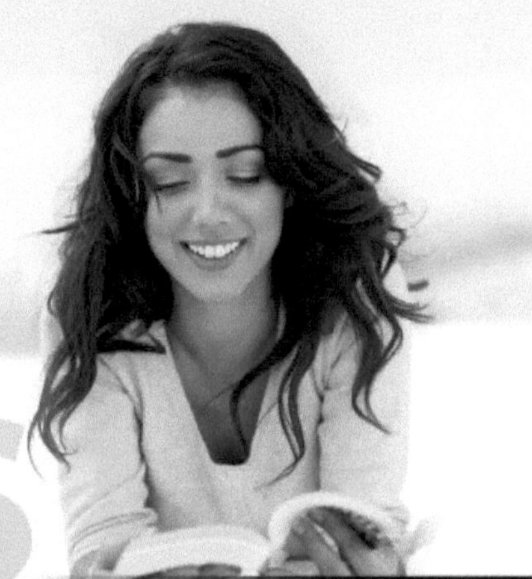

yes
I want morebooks!

Buy your books fast and straightforward online - at one of world's fastest growing online book stores! Environmentally sound due to Print-on-Demand technologies.

Buy your books online at
www.morebooks.shop

Kaufen Sie Ihre Bücher schnell und unkompliziert online – auf einer der am schnellsten wachsenden Buchhandelsplattformen weltweit! Dank Print-On-Demand umwelt- und ressourcenschonend produzi ert.

Bücher schneller online kaufen
www.morebooks.shop

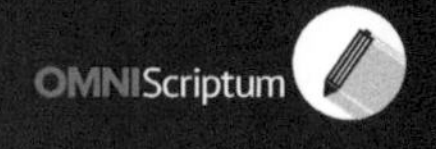

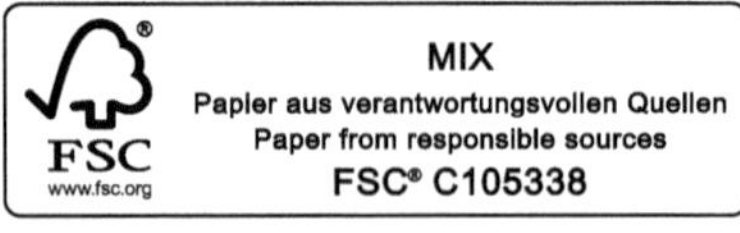

Printed by Books on Demand GmbH, Norderstedt / Germany